Table of Content

Introduction:

Welcome to "Wholesome Flavors: A Guide to Healthy and Clean Eating." In a world bustling with fast food temptations and processed snacks, it's easy to lose sight of the profound impact that mindful eating can have on our lives. This cookbook is your compass, guiding you toward a fulfilling and vibrant culinary journey that celebrates the harmonious blend of taste and nourishment.

Amid the hustle and bustle of modern life, finding the balance between satisfying your taste buds and caring for your body might seem like a daunting task. However, "Wholesome Flavors" is here to show you that healthy eating is not a sacrifice, but a celebration of the incredible bounty that nature provides.

In these pages, we'll venture beyond the confines of traditional diets and fads, embracing a philosophy that nourishes both body and soul. Each recipe is a canvas, painted with the vibrant hues of fresh produce, lean proteins, and whole grains. We'll explore a symphony of ingredients that will awaken your senses and redefine your relationship with food.

But this cookbook is more than just a collection of recipes; it's a guide to a lifestyle that empowers you to make informed choices. You'll discover the benefits of choosing ingredients that are as close to their natural state as possible, harnessing their inherent goodness to fuel your body's vitality.
The recipes within these pages aren't just meals; they're a celebration of your commitment to a healthier, happier you.

Whether you're a seasoned chef or a kitchen novice, "Wholesome Flavors" is your companion on this culinary expedition. It offers not only delectable dishes but also the knowledge and inspiration needed to craft your own culinary creations. With a focus on balance and variety, you'll find recipes that cater to different tastes, dietary preferences, and occasions.

So, tie on your apron and join us in this exploration of flavours that honour the essence of real food. Let

"Wholesome Flavors" be your inspiration, your resource, and your partner in creating meals that speak to your heart, invigorate your body, and delight your taste buds. Your journey toward a healthier, more vibrant life starts here, one wholesome bite at a time.

CHAPTER ONE:

Rise and Shine - Nutrient-Packed Breakfasts

1.   Superfood Smoothie Bowl

Start your day with a burst of energy! This colourful Superfood Smoothie Bowl is a delightful blend of antioxidant-rich berries, creamy yoghurt, and nutritious seeds. Here's how to prepare it:

Ingredients:

- 1 cup mixed berries (such as strawberries, blueberries, and raspberries), frozen or fresh
- 1 ripe banana
- 1/2 cup Greek yoghourt
- 1 tablespoon chia seeds
- 2 tablespoons granola
- Fresh mint leaves for garnish

Instructions:

1. In a blender, combine the mixed berries, banana, and Greek yoghourt. Blend until smooth and creamy.

2. Pour the smoothie into a bowl.

3. Sprinkle chia seeds and granola over the top.

4. Garnish with fresh mint leaves for a burst of freshness.

5. Grab a spoon and enjoy the vibrant flavours and textures of this nutritious bowl!

2.   Avocado and Spinach Breakfast Wrap

This savoury wrap is a quick and satisfying way to fuel your morning. Creamy avocado and nutrient-packed spinach are wrapped in a whole wheat tortilla for a portable breakfast.

Ingredients:

- 1 whole wheat tortilla
- 1 ripe avocado, sliced
- 1 cup baby spinach leaves
- 2 eggs, scrambled
- Salt and pepper to taste

Instructions:

1. Heat a non-stick skillet over medium heat.

2. Scramble the eggs in the skillet until fully cooked. Season with salt and pepper.

3. Lay the whole wheat tortilla flat on a clean surface.

4. Layer the scrambled eggs, sliced avocado, and baby spinach in the centre of the tortilla.

5. Fold in the sides of the tortilla and roll it up tightly to create a wrap.

6. Place the wrap seam-side down in the skillet and cook for a couple of minutes on each side until lightly toasted.

7. Remove from the skillet, slice in half, and savour the creamy avocado and hearty spinach in every bite.

3.   Berry Quinoa Parfait

Elevate your breakfast game with this delightful Berry Quinoa Parfait. The nutty quinoa, sweet berries, and creamy yoghourt create a harmonious blend of flavours and textures.

Ingredients:

- 1/2 cup cooked quinoa, cooled

- 1/2 cup mixed berries (strawberries, blueberries, raspberries)

- 1/2 cup Greek yoghourt

- 1 tablespoon honey or maple syrup

- 2 tablespoons chopped nuts (such as almonds or walnuts)

Instructions:

1. In a glass or jar, layer half of the cooked quinoa at the bottom.

2. Add a layer of mixed berries on top of the quinoa.

3. Drizzle a spoonful of Greek yoghourt over the berries.

4. Repeat the layers until the glass is filled.

5. Drizzle honey or maple syrup on the top layer of yoghourt.

6. Sprinkle chopped nuts for a delightful crunch.

7. Dive your spoon into the layers and experience the symphony of flavours that this parfait offers.

4.   Veggie-Packed Omelette

A Veggie-Packed Omelette is a classic breakfast choice that's customizable and nutrient-rich. Fill it with your favourite veggies for a satisfying and wholesome start to your day.

Ingredients:
- 3 eggs
- 1/4 cup bell peppers, diced
- 1/4 cup tomatoes, diced
- 1/4 cup spinach, chopped
- 1/4 cup shredded cheese (such as cheddar or feta)
- Salt and pepper to taste
- 1 teaspoon olive oil

Instructions:
1. In a bowl, whisk the eggs until well combined. Season with salt and pepper.

2. Heat olive oil in a non-stick skillet over medium heat.

3. Add diced bell peppers and tomatoes to the skillet. Sauté for a few minutes until slightly softened.

4. Pour the whisked eggs over the veggies in the skillet.

5. Allow the eggs to cook undisturbed for a minute or two until the edges set.

6. Sprinkle chopped spinach and shredded cheese evenly over one half of the omelette.

7. Gently fold the other half of the omelette over the filling.

8. Cook for another minute or until the cheese is melted and the omelette is fully cooked.

9. Slide the omelette onto a plate and enjoy the medley of veggies and cheese in each bite.

5.   Chia Seed Pudding with Fresh Fruit

Chia Seed Pudding is a versatile and nutritious breakfast option that you can prepare ahead of time. The pudding's creamy texture pairs perfectly with a medley of fresh fruit.

Ingredients:
- 3 tablespoons chia seeds
- 1 cup almond milk (or any milk of your choice)
- 1 tablespoon honey or maple syrup
- 1/2 teaspoon vanilla extract
- Fresh fruit (such as berries, kiwi, and banana) for topping

Instructions:

1. In a bowl, whisk together chia seeds, almond milk, honey or maple syrup, and vanilla extract.

2. Cover the bowl and refrigerate for at least 2 hours or overnight, allowing the chia seeds to absorb the liquid and create a pudding-like consistency.

3. Before serving, give the chia pudding a good stir to evenly distribute the seeds.

4. Spoon the chia seed pudding into serving bowls or glasses.

5. Top with a variety of fresh fruit for a burst of colour and natural sweetness.

6. Dive into the luscious chia seed pudding, savouring the delightful contrast between the creamy base and the juicy fruit topping.

These nutrient-packed breakfast recipes are just the beginning of your journey to a healthier and more vibrant lifestyle. As you indulge in these flavoursome creations, you'll discover the magic of starting your day with nourishment that awakens your senses and energises your body. Remember, each morning presents an opportunity to set a positive tone for the day ahead,

and these breakfast delights are here to inspire you on
that delicious path.

CHAPTER TWO

Wholesome Lunch Delights

6.   Mediterranean Chickpea Salad

Transport your taste buds to the shores of the Mediterranean with this vibrant and refreshing Chickpea Salad. Packed with colourful vegetables and aromatic herbs, it's a true celebration of flavours.

Ingredients:

- 1 can (15 oz) chickpeas, drained and rinsed
- 1 cup cherry tomatoes, halved
- 1 cucumber, diced
- 1/2 red onion, finely chopped
- 1/4 cup Kalamata olives, pitted and sliced
- 1/4 cup crumbled feta cheese
- 1/4 cup fresh parsley, chopped
- 2 tablespoons extra-virgin olive oil
- 2 tablespoons red wine vinegar
- Salt and pepper to taste

Instructions:

1. In a large bowl, combine chickpeas, cherry tomatoes, cucumber, red onion, olives, feta cheese, and parsley.

2. In a small bowl, whisk together olive oil and red wine vinegar to create the dressing.

3. Drizzle the dressing over the salad and toss gently to combine.

4. Season with salt and pepper to taste.

5. Allow the flavours to meld for a few minutes before serving. This vibrant salad can stand on its own as a satisfying lunch or be paired with grilled chicken or whole grain bread.

7.   Grilled Vegetable and Hummus Wrap

Elevate your lunch with this Grilled Vegetable and Hummus Wrap. It's a delightful medley of grilled veggies, creamy hummus, and a touch of tangy balsamic glaze, all wrapped in a whole wheat tortilla.

Ingredients:
  - 1 whole wheat tortilla
  - 1/2 cup hummus (store-bought or homemade)

- 1 cup mixed grilled vegetables (such as zucchini, bell peppers, and eggplant)
- 2 tablespoons balsamic glaze
- Fresh basil leaves for garnish

Instructions:

1. Lay the whole wheat tortilla flat on a clean surface.

2. Spread a generous layer of hummus over the tortilla.

3. Place the mixed grilled vegetables on top of the hummus.

4. Drizzle balsamic glaze over the vegetables.

5. Garnish with fresh basil leaves for a burst of aromatic freshness.

6. Roll up the tortilla tightly to create a wrap.

7. Slice in half and enjoy the harmonious blend of flavours and textures in each bite.

8.   Quinoa-Stuffed Bell Peppers

These Quinoa-Stuffed Bell Peppers are a delightful and wholesome lunch option. Colourful bell peppers are filled with a protein-packed quinoa stuffing, creating a balanced and satisfying meal.

Ingredients:

- 2 large bell peppers (any colour)
- 1 cup cooked quinoa
- 1/2 cup black beans, drained and rinsed
- 1/2 cup corn kernels (fresh, frozen, or canned)
- 1/4 cup diced tomatoes
- 1/4 cup shredded cheese (such as Monterey Jack or cheddar)
- 1 teaspoon chilli powder
- 1/2 teaspoon cumin
- Salt and pepper to taste
- Fresh cilantro leaves for garnish

Instructions:

1. Preheat the oven to 375°F (190°C).

2. Cut the tops off the bell peppers and remove the seeds and membranes.

3. In a bowl, combine cooked quinoa, black beans, corn, diced tomatoes, shredded cheese, chilli powder, cumin, salt, and pepper.

4. Stuff the bell peppers with the quinoa mixture, pressing down gently to pack the stuffing.

5. Place the stuffed bell peppers in a baking dish and cover with aluminium foil.

6. Bake in the preheated oven for 25-30 minutes or until the bell peppers are tender.

7. Remove the foil and bake for an additional 5 minutes to lightly brown the cheese.

8. Garnish with fresh cilantro leaves before serving. These stuffed bell peppers make a hearty and flavorful lunch that's sure to satisfy.

9.   Lentil and Kale Soup

Warm your soul with a comforting bowl of Lentil and Kale Soup. This hearty soup is brimming with protein-rich lentils, vibrant kale, and aromatic herbs.

Ingredients:

- 1 cup dried green or brown lentils, rinsed and drained
- 1 tablespoon olive oil
- 1 onion, chopped
- 2 carrots, peeled and diced
- 2 celery stalks, diced
- 3 cloves garlic, minced
- 6 cups vegetable broth
- 2 cups kale, stems removed and chopped
- 1 teaspoon dried thyme

- 1 teaspoon dried oregano

- Salt and pepper to taste

- Juice of 1 lemon

- Fresh parsley for garnish

Instructions:

1. In a large pot, heat olive oil over medium heat.

2. Add chopped onion, diced carrots, and diced celery. Sauté until the vegetables are tender.

3. Stir in minced garlic, dried thyme, and dried oregano. Cook for another minute until fragrant.

4. Add rinsed lentils and vegetable broth to the pot. Bring to a boil.

5. Reduce the heat, cover, and simmer for about 20-25 minutes or until the lentils are tender.

6. Stir in chopped kale and cook for an additional 5 minutes until the kale is wilted.

7. Season with salt, pepper, and lemon juice.

8. Ladle the soup into bowls and garnish with fresh parsley.

9. Serve this comforting lentil and kale soup with a slice of whole grain bread for a wholesome and nourishing lunch.

10.   Thai-Inspired Peanut Noodles

Indulge in the exotic flavours of Thailand with these delectable Thai-Inspired Peanut Noodles. The creamy peanut sauce coats tender noodles and colourful vegetables for a lunch that's both satisfying and flavorful.

Ingredients:

- 8 oz rice noodles, cooked according to package instructions and drained
    - 1 cup colourful bell peppers, thinly sliced
    - 1 cup shredded carrots
    - 1/2 cup edamame (cooked and shelled)
    - 1/4 cup chopped green onions
    - 1/4 cup chopped cilantro
    - 1/4 cup chopped peanuts
    - Lime wedges for serving

    For the Peanut Sauce:
    - 1/4 cup peanut butter
    - 2 tablespoons soy sauce
    - 1 tablespoon sesame oil

- 1 tablespoon rice vinegar

- 1 tablespoon honey or maple syrup

- 1 teaspoon grated fresh ginger

- 1 clove garlic, minced

- Crushed red pepper flakes (optional, for heat)

Instructions:

1. In a small bowl, whisk together all the ingredients for the peanut sauce until smooth. Adjust the flavours to your preference.

2. In a large mixing bowl, combine cooked rice noodles, sliced bell peppers, shredded carrots, edamame, chopped green onions, and chopped cilantro.

3. Pour the peanut sauce over the noodle mixture and toss to coat everything evenly.

4. Divide the Thai-inspired peanut noodles into serving bowls.

5. Sprinkle chopped peanuts over the top for added crunch.

6. Serve with lime wedges on the side for a zesty burst of flavour.

7. Delight in the harmonious blend of textures and taste in every forkful of these vibrant peanut noodles.

These Wholesome Lunch Delights are designed to nourish your body and provide you with the energy you need to conquer the day. From the Mediterranean-inspired flavours of the chickpea salad to the exotic allure of the Thai-inspired peanut noodles, these recipes celebrate the beauty of whole ingredients and creative combinations. Enjoy these lunches with the knowledge that you're making a positive choice for your well-being and indulging in meals that are as delightful as they are nutritious.

CHAPTER THREE:

Vibrant Salads and Sides

11.   Roasted Beet and Goat Cheese Salad

This Roasted Beet and Goat Cheese Salad is a masterpiece of contrasting flavours and textures. Earthy roasted beets, creamy goat cheese, and crunchy nuts come together for a salad that's as beautiful as it is delicious.

Ingredients:

- 3 medium beets, peeled and cubed
- 2 cups mixed greens (such as arugula and spinach)
- 1/4 cup crumbled goat cheese
- 1/4 cup chopped walnuts or pecans, toasted
- 2 tablespoons balsamic vinegar
- 1 tablespoon extra-virgin olive oil
- 1 teaspoon honey
- Salt and pepper to taste

Instructions:

1. Preheat the oven to 400°F (200°C).

2. Place the cubed beets on a baking sheet and drizzle with olive oil. Season with salt and pepper and toss to coat.

3. Roast the beets in the preheated oven for about 25-30 minutes, or until tender.

4. In a small bowl, whisk together balsamic vinegar, olive oil, honey, salt, and pepper to create the dressing.

5. In a large bowl, combine the roasted beets, mixed greens, crumbled goat cheese, and toasted nuts.

6. Drizzle the balsamic dressing over the salad and toss gently to combine.

7. Serve this visually stunning salad as a light and elegant side dish or add grilled chicken for a satisfying main course.

12.   Cucumber, Tomato, and Feta Salad

Embrace the essence of summer with this refreshing Cucumber, Tomato, and Feta Salad. Crisp cucumbers, juicy tomatoes, and tangy feta cheese are tossed in a light vinaigrette for a delightful side dish.

Ingredients:

- 2 cucumbers, diced
- 1 cup cherry tomatoes, halved
- 1/4 cup red onion, finely chopped
- 1/4 cup crumbled feta cheese
- 2 tablespoons fresh basil, chopped
- 2 tablespoons extra-virgin olive oil
- 1 tablespoon red wine vinegar
- Salt and pepper to taste

Instructions:

1. In a large bowl, combine diced cucumbers, halved cherry tomatoes, chopped red onion, crumbled feta cheese, and chopped fresh basil.

2. In a small bowl, whisk together extra-virgin olive oil and red wine vinegar to create the vinaigrette.

3. Drizzle the vinaigrette over the salad and toss gently to coat all the ingredients.

4. Season with salt and pepper to taste.

5. Allow the salad to marinate for a few minutes before serving. This vibrant salad complements a variety of dishes and adds a burst of colour to your table.

13. Quinoa and Mango Salad

Quinoa takes centre stage in this Quinoa and Mango Salad, paired with juicy mango, crisp vegetables, and a zesty lime dressing. It's a tropical-inspired side that's perfect for any occasion.

Ingredients:

- 1 cup cooked quinoa, cooled
- 1 ripe mango, peeled, pitted, and diced
- 1/2 red bell pepper, diced
- 1/4 cup red onion, finely chopped
- 1/4 cup fresh cilantro, chopped
- 2 tablespoons fresh lime juice
- 1 tablespoon extra-virgin olive oil
- Salt and pepper to taste

Instructions:

1. In a large bowl, combine cooked quinoa, diced mango, diced red bell pepper, chopped red onion, and chopped cilantro.

2. In a small bowl, whisk together fresh lime juice, extra-virgin olive oil, salt, and pepper to create the dressing.

3. Drizzle the dressing over the quinoa mixture and toss gently to combine.

4. Allow the flavours to meld for a few minutes before serving. This quinoa and mango salad is a burst of sunshine on your plate and a perfect accompaniment to grilled proteins or seafood.

14.   Roasted Brussels Sprouts with Balsamic Glaze

Elevate Brussels sprouts to new heights with this Roasted Brussels Sprouts with Balsamic Glaze. The caramelised sweetness of balsamic glaze complements the roasted sprouts' earthy flavour, creating a side dish that's both elegant and delicious.

Ingredients:

- 1 pound Brussels sprouts, trimmed and halved
- 2 tablespoons olive oil
- Salt and pepper to taste
- 2 tablespoons balsamic glaze
- Grated Parmesan cheese for garnish

Instructions:

1. Preheat the oven to 400°F (200°C).

2. Toss halved Brussels sprouts with olive oil, salt, and pepper in a bowl until evenly coated.

3. Spread the Brussels sprouts in a single layer on a baking sheet.

4. Roast in the preheated oven for about 20-25 minutes, stirring halfway through, until the sprouts are golden brown and crispy on the edges.

5. Drizzle balsamic glaze over the roasted Brussels sprouts and toss to coat.

6. Transfer the Brussels sprouts to a serving dish and sprinkle grated Parmesan cheese over the top.

7. Serve as a delectable side dish that brings a touch of sophistication to any meal.

15.   Sweet Potato Fries with Yogurt Dip

Indulge in the irresistible combination of Sweet Potato Fries with Yogurt Dip. Crispy baked sweet potato fries are paired with a tangy and creamy yoghourt dip for a side that's perfect for sharing.

Ingredients:

- 2 large sweet potatoes, peeled and cut into fries
- 2 tablespoons olive oil
- 1 teaspoon paprika

- 1/2 teaspoon garlic powder
- Salt and pepper to taste

For the Yogurt Dip:
- 1/2 cup Greek yoghourt
- 1 tablespoon lemon juice
- 1 tablespoon fresh dill, chopped
- Salt and pepper to taste

Instructions:

1. Preheat the oven to 425°F (220°C).

2. In a large bowl, toss sweet potato fries with olive oil, paprika, garlic powder, salt, and pepper until evenly coated.

3. Spread the sweet potato fries in a single layer on a baking sheet.

4. Bake in the preheated oven for about 25-30 minutes, flipping the fries halfway through, until they are golden and crispy.

5. While the fries are baking, prepare the yoghourt dip. In a bowl, whisk together Greek yoghourt, lemon juice, chopped fresh dill, salt, and pepper.

6. Serve the sweet potato fries hot with the creamy yoghourt dip on the side for a delightful combination of flavours and textures.

These Vibrant Salads and Sides are your invitation to explore a world of colour, freshness, and flavour. From the earthy elegance of the Roasted Beet and Goat Cheese Salad to the tropical allure of the Quinoa and Mango Salad, each dish is a celebration of the ingredients' natural beauty. Whether you're looking for a refreshing side to complement your main course or a standalone salad that steals the spotlight, these recipes will leave you craving the vibrant and wholesome goodness that they bring to your table.

CHAPTER FOUR:

Hearty Dinners with a Twist

16.   Zucchini Noodles with Pesto

Embrace a lighter take on pasta with Zucchini Noodles with Pesto. Fresh zucchini noodles are coated in vibrant basil pesto, creating a satisfying and nutritious dinner.

Ingredients:

- 4 medium zucchinis, spiralized into noodles
- 1 cup cherry tomatoes, halved
- 1/4 cup pine nuts, toasted
- 1/4 cup grated Parmesan cheese
- Fresh basil leaves for garnish

For the Basil Pesto:
- 2 cups fresh basil leaves
- 1/2 cup grated Parmesan cheese
- 1/4 cup pine nuts

- 2 cloves garlic

- 1/2 cup extra-virgin olive oil

- Salt and pepper to taste

Instructions:

1. To make the basil pesto, combine fresh basil leaves, grated Parmesan cheese, pine nuts, and garlic in a food processor. Pulse until coarsely chopped.

2. With the food processor running, slowly drizzle in the olive oil until the pesto is smooth and well combined. Season with salt and pepper to taste.

3. In a large skillet, sauté the zucchini noodles over medium heat for 2-3 minutes until they are slightly softened but still retain some crunch.

4. Toss the zucchini noodles with a generous amount of basil pesto until evenly coated.

5. Divide the zucchini noodles into serving plates.

6. Top with halved cherry tomatoes, toasted pine nuts, grated Parmesan cheese, and fresh basil leaves.

7. Serve this vibrant and flavorful dish as a light yet satisfying dinner that's sure to delight your taste buds.

17.   Baked Salmon with Lemon-Dill Sauce

Elevate your dinner with the elegance of Baked Salmon with Lemon-Dill Sauce. Tender and flaky baked salmon is complemented by a zesty lemon-dill sauce for a dish that's as impressive as it is delicious.

Ingredients:
   - 4 salmon fillets
   - 2 tablespoons olive oil
   - Salt and pepper to taste

For the Lemon-Dill Sauce:
   - 1/2 cup Greek yoghourt
   - 2 tablespoons fresh lemon juice
   - 1 tablespoon fresh dill, chopped
   - 1 teaspoon Dijon mustard
   - Salt and pepper to taste

Instructions:
   1. Preheat the oven to 375°F (190°C).

   2. Place the salmon fillets on a baking sheet. Drizzle with olive oil and season with salt and pepper.

   3. Bake in the preheated oven for about 15-20 minutes, or until the salmon flakes easily with a fork.

   4. While the salmon is baking, prepare the lemon-dill sauce. In a bowl, whisk together Greek yoghourt, fresh

lemon juice, chopped dill, Dijon mustard, salt, and pepper.

5. Serve the baked salmon fillets with a dollop of lemon-dill sauce on top.

6. Pair with your favourite roasted vegetables or a light salad for a well-rounded and nutritious dinner.

18.   Spaghetti Squash Primavera

Explore the world of vegetable-based pasta with Spaghetti Squash Primavera. Roasted spaghetti squash serves as the base for a medley of colourful sautéed vegetables and a light tomato sauce.

Ingredients:

- 1 medium spaghetti squash, halved and seeds removed
- 1 cup cherry tomatoes, halved
- 1/2 cup bell peppers, diced
- 1/2 cup zucchini, diced
- 1/4 cup red onion, finely chopped
- 2 cloves garlic, minced
- 1/4 cup grated Parmesan cheese
- Fresh basil leaves for garnish

For the Tomato Sauce:
- 1 can (14 oz) crushed tomatoes
- 2 tablespoons extra-virgin olive oil
- 1 teaspoon dried oregano
- 1/2 teaspoon dried basil
- Salt and pepper to taste

Instructions:

1. Preheat the oven to 400°F (200°C).

2. Place the spaghetti squash halves cut-side down on a baking sheet.

3. Roast in the preheated oven for about 30-40 minutes, or until the squash strands can be easily separated with a fork.

4. While the spaghetti squash is roasting, prepare the tomato sauce. In a saucepan, heat olive oil over medium heat. Add minced garlic and sauté until fragrant.

5. Stir in crushed tomatoes, dried oregano, dried basil, salt, and pepper. Simmer for a few minutes until the flavours meld.

6. In a large skillet, sauté diced bell peppers, diced zucchini, and chopped red onion until the vegetables are tender.

7. Use a fork to separate the spaghetti squash strands and add them to the skillet with the sautéed vegetables.

8. Pour the tomato sauce over the spaghetti squash and vegetables. Toss gently to combine and heat through.

9. Serve the Spaghetti Squash Primavera in the roasted squash halves or on individual plates.

10. Sprinkle grated Parmesan cheese and garnish with fresh basil leaves before serving this delightful vegetable-based pasta dish.

19.   Teriyaki Tofu Stir-Fry

Embark on a culinary adventure with this Teriyaki Tofu Stir-Fry. Marinated tofu and an array of colourful vegetables are stir-fried to perfection in a savoury and slightly sweet teriyaki sauce.

Ingredients:

- 1 block extra-firm tofu, pressed and cubed

- 2 cups mixed vegetables (such as bell peppers, broccoli, snap peas)

- 2 tablespoons vegetable oil

- 1/4 cup teriyaki sauce

- 2 tablespoons soy sauce

- 1 tablespoon honey or maple syrup

- 1 teaspoon sesame oil

- 1 teaspoon grated fresh ginger

- 2 cloves garlic, minced

- Sesame seeds and chopped green onions for garnish

Instructions:

1. In a bowl, whisk together teriyaki sauce, soy sauce, honey or maple syrup, sesame oil, grated ginger, and minced garlic to create the marinade.

2. Toss the cubed tofu in the marinade and let it marinate for at least 20 minutes.

3. In a large skillet or wok, heat vegetable oil over medium-high heat.

4. Add marinated tofu and sauté until golden and crispy on all sides. Remove from the skillet and set aside.

5. In the same skillet, add more oil if needed and stir-fry mixed vegetables until tender-crisp.

6. Return the tofu to the skillet and pour any remaining marinade over the tofu and vegetables.

7. Toss everything together and cook for another minute

or two until heated through.

8. Serve the Teriyaki Tofu Stir-Fry over cooked brown rice or quinoa.

9. Garnish with sesame seeds and chopped green onions for a touch of freshness and crunch.

20. Stuffed Bell Peppers with Quinoa and Black Beans

Delight in the wholesome goodness of Stuffed Bell Peppers with Quinoa and Black Beans. Colourful bell peppers are filled with a protein-packed quinoa and black bean stuffing, creating a satisfying and nutritious dinner.

Ingredients:
   - 4 large bell peppers (any colour)
   - 1 cup cooked quinoa
   - 1 cup black beans, drained and rinsed
   - 1 cup diced tomatoes
   - 1/2 cup shredded cheese (such as Monterey Jack or cheddar)
   - 1 teaspoon chilli powder
   - 1/2 teaspoon cumin
   - Salt and pepper to taste

- Fresh cilantro leaves for garnish

Instructions:

1. Preheat the oven to 375°F (190°C).

2. Cut the tops off the bell peppers and remove the seeds and membranes.

3. In a bowl, combine cooked quinoa, black beans, diced tomatoes, shredded cheese, chilli powder, cumin, salt, and pepper.

4. Stuff the bell peppers with the quinoa and black bean stuffing, pressing down gently to pack the filling.

5. Place the stuffed bell peppers in a baking dish and cover with aluminium foil.

6. Bake in the preheated oven for 25-30 minutes or until the bell peppers are tender.

7. Remove the foil and bake for an additional 5 minutes to lightly brown the cheese.

8. Garnish with fresh cilantro leaves before serving. These stuffed bell peppers make a hearty and flavorful dinner that's both satisfying and nourishing.

These Hearty Dinners with a Twist are an invitation to explore innovative and wholesome flavours. From the refreshing Zucchini Noodles with Pesto to the comfort of Stuffed Bell Peppers with Quinoa and Black Beans, these recipes offer a delightful twist on familiar classics. With a focus on nourishing ingredients and creative combinations, these dinners are designed to satisfy your cravings while fueling your body with the nutrients it deserves. Enjoy the journey of culinary discovery as you prepare and savour each of these hearty and delicious meals.

CHAPTER FIVE

Decadent Desserts with a Healthy Twist

21.   Dark Chocolate Avocado Mousse

Indulge your sweet tooth with this guilt-free Dark Chocolate Avocado Mousse. Creamy avocado and rich dark chocolate come together to create a luscious and satisfying dessert.

Ingredients:
- 2 ripe avocados, peeled and pitted
- 1/4 cup unsweetened cocoa powder
- 1/4 cup honey or maple syrup
- 1 teaspoon vanilla extract
- Pinch of salt
- Fresh berries for garnish

Instructions:

1. In a food processor or blender, combine ripe avocados, unsweetened cocoa powder, honey or maple syrup, vanilla extract, and a pinch of salt.

2. Blend until smooth and creamy, scraping down the sides as needed.

3. Divide the avocado mousse into serving dishes.

4. Chill in the refrigerator for at least 1 hour before serving.

5. Garnish with fresh berries before indulging in this decadent and nutritious dessert.

22.   Baked Apple with Cinnamon and Walnuts

Experience the comforting flavours of fall with this Baked Apple with Cinnamon and Walnuts. Warm, tender apples are filled with a delightful mixture of cinnamon and walnuts for a simple and wholesome treat.

Ingredients:

- 2 apples (such as Honeycrisp or Granny Smith), cored

- 2 tablespoons chopped walnuts

- 1 tablespoon honey or maple syrup

- 1/2 teaspoon ground cinnamon

- Greek yoghourt or vanilla ice cream for serving (optional)

Instructions:

1. Preheat the oven to 375°F (190°C).

2. In a bowl, combine chopped walnuts, honey or maple syrup, and ground cinnamon.

3. Fill the cored centre of each apple with the walnut mixture.

4. Place the filled apples in a baking dish.

5. Bake in the preheated oven for about 25-30 minutes, or until the apples are tender.

6. Serve the baked apples warm, with a dollop of Greek yoghourt or a scoop of vanilla ice cream, if desired.

23.   Chia Seed Chocolate Pudding

Satisfy your chocolate cravings with this Chia Seed Chocolate Pudding. Velvety cocoa and nutrient-packed chia seeds combine to create a creamy and delectable dessert.

Ingredients:

   - 1/4 cup chia seeds
   - 2 tablespoons unsweetened cocoa powder
   - 1 tablespoon honey or maple syrup
   - 1/2 teaspoon vanilla extract
   - 1 cup almond milk (or any milk of your choice)
   - Fresh berries or sliced bananas for topping

Instructions:

1. In a bowl, whisk together chia seeds, unsweetened cocoa powder, honey or maple syrup, and vanilla extract.

2. Gradually pour in almond milk while whisking to prevent clumps.

3. Continue whisking until the mixture is well combined.

4. Cover the bowl and refrigerate for at least 2 hours or overnight, allowing the chia seeds to absorb the liquid and create a pudding-like consistency.

5. Before serving, give the chia pudding a good stir to evenly distribute the seeds.

6. Spoon the chia seed chocolate pudding into serving bowls.

7. Top with fresh berries or sliced bananas for a burst of natural sweetness and colour.

8. Delight in the velvety richness of this chocolate treat that's as nourishing as it is indulgent.

24.   Frozen Banana Bites

Enjoy a cool and refreshing dessert with these Frozen Banana Bites. Slices of ripe banana are dipped in dark chocolate and frozen for a delightful treat that's perfect for satisfying your sweet tooth.

Ingredients:

- 2 ripe bananas, peeled and sliced
- 1/2 cup dark chocolate chips
- 1 teaspoon coconut oil
- Chopped nuts or shredded coconut for topping (optional)

Instructions:

1. Line a baking sheet with parchment paper.

2. Place dark chocolate chips and coconut oil in a microwave-safe bowl.

3. Microwave in 20-second intervals, stirring in between, until the chocolate is melted and smooth.

4. Dip each banana slice into the melted chocolate, allowing any excess to drip off.

5. Place the chocolate-coated banana slices on the prepared baking sheet.

6. Sprinkle chopped nuts or shredded coconut over the chocolate, if desired.

7. Place the baking sheet in the freezer and freeze for at least 1 hour, or until the chocolate is set.

8. Once frozen, transfer the banana bites to an airtight container for storage in the freezer.

9. Enjoy these Frozen Banana Bites as a delightful and guilt-free dessert whenever your sweet tooth calls.

25.   Berry Parfait with Greek Yogurt and Granola

Revel in the delightful combination of textures and flavours in this Berry Parfait with Greek Yogurt and Granola. Layers of creamy Greek yoghourt, vibrant

berries, and crunchy granola create a parfait that's as beautiful as it is delicious.

Ingredients:

- 1 cup Greek yoghourt

- 1 cup mixed berries (such as strawberries, blueberries, and raspberries)
    - 1/2 cup granola
    - Honey or maple syrup for drizzling (optional)

Instructions:

1. In serving glasses or bowls, start with a layer of Greek yoghourt.

2. Add a layer of mixed berries on top of the yoghourt.

3. Sprinkle a layer of granola over the berries.

4. Repeat the layers until the glasses or bowls are filled.

5. If desired, drizzle honey or maple syrup over the top for added sweetness.

6. Serve the Berry Parfait as a delightful and visually appealing dessert that's perfect for any occasion.

These Decadent Desserts with a Healthy Twist offer a delightful way to indulge your sweet cravings while staying true to your commitment to healthy and clean eating. From the velvety Dark Chocolate Avocado Mousse to the refreshing Frozen Banana Bites, each dessert is a testament to the creative possibilities of using nourishing ingredients. Enjoy these treats guilt-free, knowing that they not only satisfy your taste buds but also contribute to your overall well-being.

CHAPTER SIX

Quick and Energising Snacks

26.   Homemade Trail Mix

Fuel your body with the goodness of nuts, seeds, and dried fruits in this Homemade Trail Mix. Create your perfect blend of energy-boosting ingredients for a satisfying and portable snack.

Ingredients:

- 1 cup mixed nuts (such as almonds, walnuts, cashews)

- 1/2 cup dried fruits (such as raisins, dried cranberries, apricots)

- 1/4 cup seeds (such as pumpkin seeds, sunflower seeds)

- 1/4 cup dark chocolate chips or cacao nibs

Instructions:

1. In a bowl, mix together mixed nuts, dried fruits, seeds, and dark chocolate chips.

2. Divide the trail mix into individual portion-sized containers or snack bags.

3. Grab a handful whenever you need a quick and energising snack that's perfect for on-the-go.

27.   Greek Yogurt and Berry Parfait

Experience a burst of flavour and protein with this Greek Yogurt and Berry Parfait. Creamy Greek yoghourt is layered with vibrant berries and a sprinkle of nuts for a satisfying and nutritious snack.

Ingredients:

- 1 cup Greek yoghourt

- 1/2 cup mixed berries (such as strawberries, blueberries, raspberries)

- 2 tablespoons chopped nuts (such as almonds or walnuts)

- Honey or maple syrup for drizzling (optional)

Instructions:

1. In a glass or small bowl, start with a layer of Greek yoghourt.

2. Add a layer of mixed berries on top of the yoghourt.

3. Sprinkle chopped nuts over the berries.

4. Repeat the layers until the glass or bowl is filled.

5. If desired, drizzle honey or maple syrup over the top for added sweetness.

6. Enjoy the Greek Yogurt and Berry Parfait as a refreshing and protein-packed snack.

28.   Apple Slices with Nut Butter

Elevate the classic combination of apples and nut butter for a delightful and satisfying snack. Crisp apple slices are paired with creamy nut butter for a balanced and nourishing treat.

Ingredients:

- 1 apple, sliced

- 2 tablespoons nut butter (such as almond butter, peanut butter)

Instructions:

1. Slice the apple into thin wedges.

2. Dip each apple slice into nut butter and enjoy the delightful contrast of textures and flavours.

29.   Crispy Roasted Chickpeas

Experience the addictive crunch of Crispy Roasted Chickpeas. These protein-packed snacks are seasoned and roasted to perfection for a savoury and satisfying treat.

Ingredients:

- 1 can (15 oz) chickpeas, drained, rinsed, and patted dry
- 1 tablespoon olive oil
- 1 teaspoon paprika
- 1/2 teaspoon cumin
- 1/4 teaspoon garlic powder
- Salt and pepper to taste

Instructions:

1. Preheat the oven to 400°F (200°C).

2. In a bowl, toss chickpeas with olive oil, paprika, cumin, garlic powder, salt, and pepper.

3. Spread the chickpeas in a single layer on a baking sheet.

4. Roast in the preheated oven for about 20-25 minutes, shaking the pan occasionally, until the chickpeas are crispy and golden.

5. Allow the roasted chickpeas to cool before enjoying this protein-packed and satisfying snack.

30.   Veggie Sticks with Hummus

Elevate your snack game with Veggie Sticks and Hummus. Crisp and colourful vegetable sticks are paired with creamy hummus for a nutritious and flavorful snack.

Ingredients:

- Assorted vegetable sticks (such as carrots, cucumber, bell peppers, celery)
- Hummus for dipping

Instructions:

1. Wash and cut the vegetables into stick shapes.

2. Serve the vegetable sticks with a bowl of hummus for dipping.

3. Enjoy the combination of crunchy vegetables and creamy hummus for a satisfying and nutrient-packed snack.

These Quick and Energising Snacks are designed to keep you fueled and satisfied throughout the day. Whether you're in need of a boost between meals or a bite to power you through a busy afternoon, these snacks offer a blend of flavours, textures, and nutrients that nourish both your body and mind. From the convenience of Homemade Trail Mix to the freshness of Veggie Sticks with Hummus, each snack is a testament to the delicious and healthful possibilities of mindful snacking.

CHAPTER SEVEN

Refreshing Beverages and Smoothies

31. Green Goddess Smoothie

Start your day with a burst of nutrients in the form of a Green Goddess Smoothie. Packed with leafy greens, fruits, and a touch of sweetness, this smoothie is a vibrant and energising way to kick-start your morning.

Ingredients:
- 1 cup spinach or kale leaves
- 1/2 banana, frozen
- 1/2 cup pineapple chunks, frozen
- 1/2 cup almond milk (or any milk of your choice)
- 1/2 cup water
- 1 tablespoon chia seeds (optional)
- 1 teaspoon honey or maple syrup (optional)

Instructions:

1. In a blender, combine spinach or kale leaves, frozen banana, frozen pineapple chunks, almond milk, water, chia seeds (if using), and honey or maple syrup (if desired).

2. Blend until smooth and creamy, adding more water if needed to reach your desired consistency.

3. Pour the Green Goddess Smoothie into a glass and enjoy the refreshing and nourishing flavours.

Berry Blast Smoothie

Quench your thirst and indulge in the sweetness of summer with a Berry Blast Smoothie. A medley of colourful berries and a splash of citrus create a delightful and antioxidant-rich beverage.

Ingredients:

- 1/2 cup mixed berries (such as strawberries, blueberries, raspberries)
- 1/2 banana, frozen
- 1/2 cup orange juice
- 1/2 cup water
- 1 tablespoon Greek yoghourt (optional)
- Fresh mint leaves for garnish

Instructions:

1. In a blender, combine mixed berries, frozen banana, orange juice, water, and Greek yoghourt (if using).

2. Blend until smooth and well combined.

3. Pour the Berry Blast Smoothie into a glass and garnish with fresh mint leaves.

4. Sip and savour the vibrant flavours of this refreshing and vitamin-packed beverage.

33. Coconut Water and Pineapple Cooler

Transport yourself to a tropical paradise with this Coconut Water and Pineapple Cooler. Hydrating coconut water and tangy pineapple create a revitalising and naturally sweetened drink.

Ingredients:

- 1 cup coconut water
- 1/2 cup pineapple chunks
- 1/4 cup fresh lime juice
- Mint sprigs for garnish

Instructions:

1. In a blender, combine coconut water, pineapple chunks, and fresh lime juice.

2. Blend until the pineapple is fully pureed and the mixture is well combined.

3. Pour the Coconut Water and Pineapple Cooler into a glass.

4. Garnish with mint sprigs for a touch of freshness and visual appeal.

5. Sip and enjoy the tropical flavours of this rejuvenating beverage.

34.   Iced Green Tea with Citrus

Stay refreshed and invigorated with a glass of Iced Green Tea with Citrus. Green tea is infused with the bright flavours of citrus for a cool and revitalising drink.

Ingredients:
- 2 green tea bags
- 4 cups water
- Slices of lemon, lime, and orange
- Fresh basil or mint leaves for garnish

Instructions:

1. Bring 4 cups of water to a boil. Remove from heat and add green tea bags.

2. Steep the green tea for about 3-4 minutes, then remove the tea bags and allow the tea to cool to room temperature.

3. Once cooled, refrigerate the green tea until chilled.

4. Fill glasses with ice and add slices of lemon, lime, and orange.

5. Pour the chilled green tea over the ice and citrus slices.

6. Garnish with fresh basil or mint leaves for a burst of aroma and flavour.

7. Sip and savour the cooling and invigorating Iced Green Tea with Citrus.

35.   Cucumber Mint Refresher

Quench your thirst with the light and revitalising flavours of a Cucumber Mint Refresher. Crisp cucumber and fragrant mint combine to create a hydrating and rejuvenating drink.

Ingredients:
   - 1 cucumber, peeled and sliced
   - 1/4 cup fresh mint leaves
   - 4 cups water
   - Slices of lemon for garnish

Instructions:

1. In a pitcher, combine cucumber slices, fresh mint leaves, and water.

2. Refrigerate the pitcher for at least 1 hour to allow the flavours to infuse.

3. Fill glasses with ice and pour the Cucumber Mint Refresher over the ice.

4. Garnish with slices of lemon for an extra burst of freshness.

5. Sip and enjoy the soothing and hydrating qualities of this revitalising beverage.

These Refreshing Beverages and Smoothies offer a delightful way to stay hydrated and invigorated throughout the day. Whether you're seeking a vibrant and nutrient-packed start to your morning or a cool and rejuvenating sip to quench your thirst, these drinks provide a range of flavours and benefits. From the Green Goddess Smoothie to the Cucumber Mint Refresher, each beverage is a testament to the creative possibilities of incorporating wholesome ingredients into your daily hydration routine.